FAT TO FIT

FAT TO FIT

*Transform Your Body,
Transform Your Life*

CASSIDY SILVERWOOD

QuantumQuill Press

CONTENTS

Introduction

Welcome to "Fat to Fit: Change Your Body, Change Your Life," an aide planned to change what you look like, yet to change how you feel, think, and draw in with your general surroundings. This book is your sidekick on an excursion from understanding the mind boggling elements of your body to dominating the psychological and close to home parts of supporting a solid way of life. Whether you're worn out on handy solutions that don't stand the test of time or feeling overpowered by clashing wellbeing counsel, this guide means to enlighten a make way through the commotion, grounded in science and individual experience.

What You Will Realize:

•The Underpinnings of Weight The executives: Understanding the organic, mental, and ecological elements adding to weight gain and misfortune.

•Wholesome Insight: Moving past weight control plans to maintainable dietary patterns that feed and fulfill.

•Practice Fundamentals: Making an activity routine that is pleasant, compelling, and customized to your life.

•Close to home and Mental Prosperity: Strategies to encourage an outlook that upholds your actual objectives, incorporating managing pressure, building strength, and embracing change.

•Way of life Change: Pragmatic guidance for incorporating sound propensities into your day to day existence, guaranteeing enduring change.

An Individual Story:

Allow me to share a story that repeats the encounters of many, including my own. Sarah, a companion and motivation, set out on her fat-to-fit venture feeling crushed by long stretches of bombed consumes less calories and transient exercise center participations. Her advancement came not from finding a mystery diet or a supernatural occurrence exercise yet from a crucial change in how she might interpret wellbeing and prosperity. Sarah figured out how to pay attention to her body, to feed it with appropriate sustenance, draw in it in active work since it was pleasant, and in particular, to regard it. This book draws on stories like Sarah's and the furthest down the line examination to direct you through a comparable change.

A Comprehensive Methodology:

This excursion isn't exclusively about shedding pounds; it's tied in with building a daily existence where wellbeing and bliss are entwined. Our methodology is all encompassing, tending to the physical as well as the profound and mental elements of change. About making a way of life is reasonable, pleasant, and enhancing.

Setting out on this excursion requires mental fortitude, responsibility, and a receptive outlook. As you turn these pages, I welcome you to connect profoundly, question unreservedly, and embrace the progressions that lie ahead. Together, we'll investigate the study of changing your body as well as the specialty of changing your life.

1

Understanding Your Body

Chapter 1: The Science of Weight Gain

Understanding the science behind weight gain is the most vital phase in dominating your body's exceptional elements. This part demystifies the natural cycles that add to weight gain and sets the establishment for informed decisions all through your change process.

Key Ideas:

•Energy Equilibrium: At its center, weight the board spins around the energy balance condition; calories consumed versus calories exhausted. In any case, this basic condition is impacted by a heap of variables including hereditary qualities, digestion, hormonal controls, and way of life factors.

•Digestion: Your digestion assumes a urgent part in how your body uses energy. We'll investigate the elements that influence metabolic rate and how you can impact them.

•Hormonal Impact: Chemicals like insulin, leptin, and ghrelin essentially influence craving, fat capacity, and yearning signals. Understanding these can help in overseeing desires and keeping up with energy levels.

•Mental Elements: Stress, rest, and close to home prosperity are profoundly entwined with weight gain. An investigate the mental perspectives offers bits of knowledge into careful eating, stress the board, and profound strength.

•Wholesome Effect: Not all calories are made equivalent. The nature of your calorie admission influences how your body processes food, impacts hormonal reactions, and at last effects weight gain.

Goals:

Toward the finish of this section, you'll have a complete comprehension of the variables adding to weight gain. This information will enable you to arrive at informed conclusions about nourishment, exercise, and way of life changes that line up with your body's necessities.

Important point:

Getting a handle on the study of weight gain enlightens the way to powerful weight the board. With this getting it, you're better prepared to explore the excursion ahead, settling on decisions that lead to a fitter body as well as to a better, more energetic life.

In the following area, we'll dig into "The Brain research of Eating," investigating how our contemplations, feelings, and ways of behaving impact our dietary patterns and how to outfit this comprehension for good change.

Chapter 2: The Psychology of Eating

Jumping further into the excursion of change, we experience a perspective frequently neglected at this point crucial in accomplishing enduring change: the brain science of eating. This part investigates the complex connection between our brains and our dietary patterns, offering bits of knowledge into how mental variables impact our food decisions and systems for outfitting this comprehension to encourage better associations with food.

Grasping Profound Eating:

•The Profound Association with Food: Large numbers of us go to nourishment for solace, stress help, or as a prize. Disentangling the profound bonds we structure with food is vital in understanding our dietary patterns.

•Distinguishing Triggers: Perceiving the close to home and situational triggers that lead to unfortunate eating designs is the most vital move toward change. This incorporates pressure, weariness, trouble, and social impacts.

•Procedures for Change: Reasonable exhortation on dealing with profound triggers, like care strategies, journaling, and laying out new, sound survival techniques.

Careful Eating:

•The Idea of Care: Prologue to careful eating as an act of being available and completely drew in with the eating experience, assisting with working on the relationship with food.

•Advantages of Careful Eating: How careful eating can prompt better piece control, expanded delight in food, and a more profound comprehension of yearning and satiety signs.

•Commonsense Tips for Careful Eating: Straightforward activities to integrate care into your feasts, including eating gradually, killing interruptions, and paying attention to your body's appetite signals.

The Job of Propensities and Climate:

•Shaping and Getting out from under Propensities: Experiences into how dietary patterns are framed and the nervous system science behind propensity change. Systems for making new, good dieting ways of behaving.

•Natural Impacts: Looking at what our environmental elements mean for our eating decisions, from the design of our kitchens to the organization we continue during dinners. Ways to establish a climate that upholds smart dieting propensities.

Mental Techniques for Conquering Obstructions:

•Managing Desires: Understanding the mental premise of desires and techniques for overseeing them without hardship.

•Building a Positive Mental self view: How to develop a positive relationship with your body and food, creating some distance from culpability and self-analysis toward acknowledgment and inspiration.

•The Significance of Self-Empathy: Embracing self-sympathy as an instrument for conquering misfortunes and cultivating a solid, feasible way to deal with eating and wellness.

Targets:

Toward the finish of this part, perusers will acquire a significant comprehension of the mental perspectives that impact eating ways of behaving. Outfitted with this information, you'll be prepared to pursue careful decisions that line up with your wellbeing objectives, comprehend and deal with your desires, and eventually, foster a better and really fulfilling relationship with food.

Action item:

The brain research of eating is a complicated snare of feelings, propensities, and ecological elements. By digging into and understanding these viewpoints, you leave on an essential step towards enduring wellbeing and health, where food turns into a wellspring of sustenance and satisfaction, as opposed to a landmark for control.

As we push ahead, the following section, "Nourishment Rudiments," will supplement this mental foundation with useful dietary information, guaranteeing you have every one of the instruments required for a comprehensive change.

Chapter 3: Nutrition Basics

As we proceed with our excursion towards change, establishing ourselves in the rudiments of sustenance is fundamental. Understanding what energizes our bodies best is basic to any enduring change in our wellbeing and wellness. This part demystifies nourishment, giving clear and noteworthy direction on pursuing informed food decisions that help your change objectives.

The Structure Blocks of Sustenance:

•Macronutrients: An outline of sugars, proteins, and fats — the essential wellsprings of energy for the body. Become familiar with the jobs they play in basicphysical processes, the amount you really want, and the best hotspots for each.

•Micronutrients: Digging into nutrients and minerals, the fundamental supplements that assist with forestalling sickness and keep up with ideal wellbeing. An aide on the best way to integrate various supplements into your eating routine.

•Water: Frequently neglected, water is essential for virtually every basicphysical process. Investigate the significance of hydration, the amount you ought to drink day to day, and the indications of parchedness.

Understanding Food Marks:

•Translating Names: An introduction on the best way to peruse and comprehend food marks, going with it simpler to pursue sound choices and stay away from stowed away sugars, fats, and sodium.

•Reality with regards to Added substances: An investigation of food added substances, what they are, their potential wellbeing effects, and how to distinguish them in your food.

Dietary Examples for Wellbeing:

•Eating Examples: An assessment of different eating designs, including Mediterranean, plant-based, and irregular fasting, featuring the advantages and contemplations of each.

•Redoing Your Eating regimen: Ways to fit these dietary examples to accommodate your way of life, inclinations, and wholesome necessities, guaranteeing manageability and happiness.

Arranging and Planning Quality Dinners:

•Feast Arranging Rudiments: Procedures for arranging sound, adjusted dinners that help your wellness objectives, save time, and decrease food squander.

•Sound Cooking Procedures: A manual for cooking strategies that protect supplements and flavor while limiting unfortunate fats and added substances.

•Shrewd Nibbling: Thoughts for nutritious bites that can fulfill hunger between dinners without crashing your advancement.

Sustenance Legends and Misguided judgments:

•Busting Normal Legends: Tending to inescapable sustenance fantasies, giving proof based data to explain disarray around themes, for example, carbs, fats, and diet crazes.

•Supplements: The job of enhancements in a fair eating regimen, when they may be required, and the dangers related with abuse.

Targets:

Toward the finish of this part, you will have a strong comprehension of healthful standards, empowering you to settle on informed conclusions about what you eat. This information will act as the establishment for the dietary changes you'll carry out on your way to becoming fit.

Focal point:

Great sustenance isn't about severe dietary restrictions or denying yourself of the food sources you love. Rather, it's tied in with feeling perfect, having more energy, working on your standpoint, and balancing out your state of mind. With the rudiments of sustenance in your tool compartment, you're prepared to make an eating routine that is custom-made to your body's requirements, tastes, and objectives.

2

Preparing for Change

Setting out on a remarkable journey from fat to fit requires some different option from getting a handle on your body and the norms of food; it demands a status for change. Preparing mentally and earnestly for this journey is crucial. This piece of the book is focused on furnishing you with the gadgets and viewpoint critical to set yourself up in a decent way.

Area 4: Characterizing Reasonable Targets

Setting viable, feasible goals is the groundwork of any productive change. This part guides you through distinctive your objectives, making a game plan that lines up with your lifestyle, and setting yourself up in a way for plausible change.

Figuring out True Setting:

•The Meaning of Reasonable Goals: Examine the reason why spreading out plausible targets is essential for motivation and long stretch accomplishment. Sort out the qualification among longing and doable targets.

•S.M.A.R.T Targets: Preface to the S.M.A.R.T (Unequivocal, Quantifiable, Reachable, Appropriate, Time-bound) objective setting structure. Sort out some way to apply this procedure to your health and prosperity objectives.

Making Your Own Layout:

•Looking over Your Early phase: A manual for looking at your continuous genuine prosperity, lifestyle, and groundwork for change. This assessment will go about as the foundation for your goal setting process.

•Long stretch versus Transient Targets: Sort out some way to counterbalance your fast focuses with your comprehensive, long stretch objectives. Ways of isolating your fundamental goal into additional humble, more reasonable accomplishments.

•Planning Targets into Your Lifestyle: Procedures for making your goals a trademark piece of your regular day to day plan, ensuring they supplement rather than battle with your ongoing commitments and obligations.

Motivation and Obligation:

•Finding Your Why: Exercises to help you with revealing the more significant clarifications for your desire to change, working on your motivation.

•Obligation Parts: The occupation of obligation in genuine achievement, including self-enrollments, progress following, and tracking down liability accessories or social occasions.

•Changing Targets For a really long time: Understanding that your cycle could anticipate that you should reconsider and change your goals. Sort out some way to stay versatile and open to your headway and troubles.

Beating Obstructions:

•Anticipating Troubles: Perceiving potential diversions to your targets and anticipating the most ideal way to overcome them.

•Adaptability Building: Making mental and up close and personal solidarity to investigate hardships and keep on pushing ahead.

Objectives:

Around the completion of this part, you will have set individual, reasonable targets that reflect your desires and status for change.

You'll be equipped with strategies for staying aware of motivation, ensuring liability, and changing your strategy dependent upon the situation.

Thing to do:

Viable goal setting isn't just about describing what you want to achieve; it's connected to making an aide for your journey, complete with accomplishments, genuinely strong organizations, and crisis blueprints. With clear, attainable targets, you're not just yearning for change; you're successfully moving towards it.

Chapter 5: Mental Preparation for Change

In the wake of defining sensible objectives, the following urgent move toward your change process includes setting up your psyche for the progressions ahead. Mental planning is tied in with developing an outlook that embraces change, beats difficulties, and supports inspiration long term. This part gives methodologies and experiences to intellectually prepare for the groundbreaking way from fat to fit.

Developing a Development Outlook:

•Figuring out Mentalities: Prologue to the idea of fixed versus development attitudes and how they impact our capacity to change and adjust.

•Fostering a Development Mentality: Useful ways to cultivate an outlook that embraces difficulties, gains from disappointments, and considers work to be the way to dominance.

•The Force of Conviction: What trusting in your capacity to change can altogether mean for your change process. Procedures for supporting positive convictions about yourself and your true capacity.

Embracing Change:

•The Brain research of Progress: Investigate how people answer change and the close to home stages you could insight during your change.

•Planning for Close to home Highs and lows: Devices for dealing with the profound parts of progress, including pressure, dread, and snapshots of uncertainty.

•Remaining Adaptable: The significance of versatility in your excursion, staying open to changing your methodologies, objectives, and strategies as you progress.

Building Mental and Profound Flexibility:

•Flexibility Preparing: Methods for building versatility, including pressure the executives, positive reasoning, and profound guideline.

•Gaining from Difficulties: Having a significant impact on your viewpoint on misfortunes, seeing them as learning open doors as opposed to disappointments.

•Keeping up with Energy: Procedures for keeping yourself spurred, in any event, when progress appears to be slow or challenges emerge.

Representation and Positive Symbolism:

•The Job of Perception: How envisioning your prosperity can improve your inspiration and the probability of accomplishing your objectives.

•Rehearsing Representation: Bit by bit manual for fostering a perception work on, integrating it into your everyday daily schedule for greatest advantage.

Establishing a Steady Mental Climate:

•Encircling Yourself with Energy: The effect of your social and instructive climate on your mentality. Ways to develop a steady, positive climate.

•Care and Reflection: Consolidating care practices to upgrade center, decrease pressure, and further develop your profound prosperity.

Targets:

Toward the finish of this section, you'll be outfitted with the psychological devices and procedures expected to move toward your change with certainty, strength, and an uplifting perspective. You'll comprehend the mental parts of progress and how to successfully explore them.

Focus point:

Mental arrangement is essentially as significant as actual status in your change process. By fostering a strong mentality, embracing change, and building flexibility, you're making way for an effective and manageable change. With your psyche arranged for the difficulties and wins ahead, you're one bit nearer to accomplishing your fat-to-fit objectives.

Chapter 6: Building a Support System

Leaving on a change venture from fat to fit is a profoundly private undertaking, yet the significance of a strong climate couldn't possibly be more significant. This section digs into the meaning of making a powerful emotionally supportive network, offering viable guidance on the best way to encircle yourself with the right blend of consolation, responsibility, and mastery to drive you toward your objectives.

Grasping the Job of an Emotionally supportive network:

•The Significance of Help: Investigate how having an organization of steady people and assets can upgrade inspiration, give responsibility, and proposition close to home comfort during testing times.

•Sorts of Help: Distinguishing various types of help — profound, educational, and instrumental — and the interesting advantages each brings to your excursion.

Making Your Encouraging group of people:

•Loved ones: Methodologies for enrolling the help of close private connections. Ways to convey your objectives and needs really to guarantee their help lines up with your excursion.

•Wellness and Wellbeing Experts: The job of expert help, including fitness coaches, nutritionists, and advisors, in giving master direction and responsibility.

•Local area and Friend Backing: Utilizing the force of local area through internet based discussions, neighborhood wellness gatherings, or weight reduction support gatherings. The advantages of interfacing with peers who share comparable objectives and difficulties.

Exploring Difficulties inside Your Emotionally supportive network:

•Managing Absence of Help: How to oversee circumstances where your quick circle may not comprehend or uphold your change objectives. Procedures for tracking down help beyond your nearby climate.

•Defining Limits: The significance of defining solid limits with allies to keep up with your concentration and stay balanced or adverse impacts.

•Looking for Proficient Assistance While Required: Perceiving when it's gainful to look for the assistance of psychological well-being experts to explore close to home barricades or dietary issues.

Amplifying the Advantage of Your Emotionally supportive network:

•Dynamic Cooperation: Being a functioning individual from your encouraging group of people by offering consolation, sharing assets, and taking part in bunch exercises or conversations.

•Responsibility Systems: Setting up ordinary registrations with your encouraging group of people to examine progress, misfortunes, and acclimations to your arrangement.

•Observing Achievements Together: Perceiving and praising accomplishments with your encouraging group of people to cultivate a feeling of local area and shared achievement.

Goals:

Toward the finish of this section, you will have the instruments and systems important to fabricate a steady organization that lines up with your change objectives. You'll comprehend how to really convey your requirements, put down stopping points, and draw in with your emotionally supportive network to amplify its advantages.

Focus point:

A strong emotionally supportive network is a basic part of any effective change venture. Via cautiously constructing and sustaining this organization, you guarantee that you have the close to home, educational, and instrumental help expected to explore the way

from fat to fit. With a solid underpinning of help, you're better prepared to confront difficulties, celebrate triumphs, and support your
change over the long haul.

3

The Transformation Journey

Now that you've laid the basis with figuring out your body, getting ready intellectually, and building an emotionally supportive network, now is the ideal time to leave on the center of your change process. This piece of the book centers around noteworthy stages and procedures for transforming your objectives into the real world, beginning with sustenance, one of the most basic parts of any weight reduction venture.

Chapter 7: Nutrition for Weight Loss

Powerful nourishment isn't just about eating less; it's tied in with eating shrewd. This part plunges profound into how to upgrade your eating regimen for weight reduction, guaranteeing that you fuel your body with the right supplements while making a calorie shortfall in a solid and economical way.

Standards of Weight reduction Sustenance:

•Calorie deficiency: Grasping the major guideline of weight reduction — consuming less calories than you consume — and how to accomplish it without undermining your wellbeing.

•Macronutrient Equilibrium: The job of proteins, fats, and starches in weight reduction. Instructions to adjust these macronutrients to help fat misfortune, protect bulk, and keep up with energy levels.

•Supplement Thickness: Zeroing in on food sources that are high in supplements yet low in calories to upgrade satiety and sustenance. The significance of entire food sources over handled choices.

Making a Weight reduction Eating Plan:

•Customized Sustenance: Fitting your eating intend to accommodate your way of life, inclinations, and explicit wholesome requirements. Contemplations for various dietary inclinations and limitations.

•Feast Timing and Recurrence: Investigating the effect of dinner timing and recurrence on weight reduction, including procedures like irregular fasting and the discussion around eating late around evening time.

•Segment Control: Methods for overseeing segment sizes to abstain from indulging while at the same time guaranteeing fulfillment and dietary ampleness.

Defeating Healthful Difficulties:

•Exploring Social Circumstances: Methodologies for adhering to your eating plan during get-togethers, occasions, and feasting out.

•Managing Desires and Profound Eating: Reasonable ways to oversee desires and close to home eating triggers, building up the mental techniques canvassed in before parts.

•Going with Supportable Decisions: How to make smart dieting a feasible piece of your way of life, including tips for shopping for food, dinner preparing, and adjusting recipes.

Supplementation and Weight reduction:

•The Job of Enhancements: A proof based see supplements usually utilized for weight reduction, their possible advantages, and impediments.

•Normal Enhancements versus Manufactured: Grasping the distinction and picking supplements carefully, if necessary, in view of wellbeing and dietary objectives.

Targets:

Toward the finish of this part, you'll have an extensive comprehension of how to change your eating regimen for successful weight reduction. You'll be outfitted with systems for making a fair, supplement rich eating plan that upholds your weight reduction objectives while being versatile to your way of life.

Focus point:

Nourishment for weight reduction is tied in with making educated, careful food decisions that line up with your body's necessities and your weight reduction objectives. By zeroing in on supplement thick food varieties, overseeing segments, and understanding the equilibrium of macronutrients, you're making way for an effective and feasible change.

Chapter 8: Exercise Essentials

Practice is a mainstay of wellbeing and a vital part of any change venture. Besides the fact that it helps with weight reduction, however it additionally works on cardiovascular wellbeing, supports state of mind, and upgrades by and large prosperity. This part centers around laying out an economical, compelling activity routine that supplements your nourishing endeavors and speeds up your excursion from fat to fit.

Grasping the Job of Practice in Weight reduction:

•Caloric Consume and Metabolic Rate: What various sorts of activity mean for calorie consumption and impact your basal metabolic rate over the long run.

•Bulk and Fat Misfortune: The significance of protecting and fabricating bulk for its metabolic advantages and how it adds to a more conditioned appearance as you lose fat.

•Exercise and Craving: A gander at what actual work means for yearning and completion signs, and systems for overseeing post-practice hunger.

Making a Reasonable Activity Program:

•Cardiovascular Activity: The advantages of vigorous activity for heart wellbeing and fat misfortune, including suggestions for recurrence, term, and power. Models incorporate strolling, running, cycling, and swimming.

•Strength Preparing: How opposition preparing upholds weight reduction, safeguards bulk, and increments strength. Direction on consolidating bodyweight works out, free loads, and machines into your daily practice.

•Adaptability and Versatility: The job of adaptability and portability practices in forestalling injury, further developing execution, and supporting in general actual wellbeing. Prologue to rehearses like yoga and extending schedules.

Beginning Your Activity Process:

•Surveying Your Wellness Level: Rules for assessing your ongoing wellness level and laying out proper activity objectives.

•Moderate Over-burden: The guideline of steadily expanding the requests on your body to keep gaining ground, including how to execute this methodology securely.

•Assortment and Satisfaction: The significance of integrating different activities to keep your routine connecting with and agreeable, lessening the gamble of burnout.

Beating Activity Boundaries:

•Using time effectively: Systems for squeezing exercise into a bustling timetable, including short, powerful exercises and integrating active work into day to day schedules.

•Inspiration and Responsibility: Methods for remaining spurred, following advancement, and utilizing your emotionally supportive network to keep you responsible.

•Managing Mishaps: How to explore normal activity difficulties, like levels, wounds, and loss of inspiration, and methodologies for refocusing.

Security and Injury Anticipation:

•Warm-Up and Chill Off: The significance of heating up before exercise and chilling off subsequently to forestall injury and further develop practice execution.

•Paying attention to Your Body: Perceiving the distinction between ordinary activity distress and potential injury torment. Ways to answer your body's signs.

Targets:

Toward the finish of this part, you will have a strong comprehension of how to make a decent, compelling activity program that suits your wellness level, inclinations, and objectives. You'll be ready to coordinate actual work into your change process in a manner that is pleasant, manageable, and helpful for weight reduction and by and large wellbeing.

Action item:

Practice isn't simply an instrument for weight reduction; it's a training for deep rooted wellbeing and prosperity. By finding exercises you appreciate and zeroing in on assortment, movement, and consistency, you set the establishment for a fit, dynamic way of life that upholds your change objectives and improves your personal satisfaction.

Chapter 9: Lifestyle Changes for Lasting Fitness

Accomplishing enduring wellness rises above diet and exercise; it's tied in with coordinating solid propensities into each feature of your life. This section centers around exhaustive way of life changes that help your change process, guaranteeing the outcomes you accomplish are supportable over the long haul. About developing a way of life normally lines up with wellbeing and prosperity, making wellness a consistent piece of your ordinary presence.

Laying out a Sound Daily schedule:

•Consistency Over Flawlessness: The significance of predictable, day to day propensities over inconsistent flawlessness. Methodologies for building a standard that integrates smart dieting, ordinary active work, and satisfactory rest.

•Rest and Recuperation: Figuring out the basic job of snooze weight reduction, muscle recuperation, and in general wellbeing. Ways to further develop rest quality and establishing a relaxing climate.

•Stress The board: Methods for overseeing pressure, which can in any case subvert your wellness objectives. Incorporates rehearses like care, reflection, and time usage methodologies.

Integrating Active work into Day to day existence:

•Past Organized Exercise: Tracking down valuable open doors for development over the course of the day, like using the stairwell, strolling or trekking for short drives, and standing work areas.

•Dynamic Diversion: Empowering commitment in sporting exercises that advance wellness as a result, such as climbing, moving, or group activities.

Sustenance as a Way of life:

•Careful Eating Works on: Proceeding with the act of careful eating by paying attention to your body's yearning and completion signals, and getting a charge out of feasts without interruption.

•Smart dieting Out: Exploring eatery menus and social eating without wrecking your nourishment objectives. Figuring out how to go with better decisions while feasting out.

•Preparing and Dinner Arrangement: The advantages of getting ready feasts at home, including command over fixings, segment sizes, and the healthy benefit of your dinners. Basic methodologies for feast arranging and prep to accommodate your bustling timetable.

Feasible Propensities for Long haul Achievement:

•Objective Reconsideration and Transformation: Occasionally rethinking and changing your objectives to mirror what is happening, accomplishments, and yearnings.

•Long lasting Getting the hang of: Remaining informed about wellbeing and wellness to adjust your way of life to arising exploration and individual experiences consistently.

•Local area and Social Help: Keeping up with and growing your encouraging group of people to incorporate people who share your obligation to a sound way of life.

Defeating Deterrents to Way of life Change:

•Natural and Social Difficulties: Systems for managing conditions and group environments that may not help your wellbeing objectives.

•Keeping up with Inspiration: Keeping the fire of inspiration alive through setting new difficulties, commending triumphs, and helping yourself to remember your "why."

Targets:

Toward the finish of this section, you will be furnished with a thorough arrangement of systems for coordinating wellness into your way of life such that feels regular and practical. You'll have the instruments to accomplish as well as keep up with your change over the long haul.

Important point:

Enduring wellness isn't an objective however an approach to everyday life. About settling on decisions consistently line up with your wellbeing objectives and adjusting your current circumstance to help these decisions. With the way of life changes illustrated in this part, you're prepared to embrace a day to day existence where wellness and prosperity are vital to your everyday presence, guaranteeing the life span of your change.

4

Overcoming Challenges

The way from fat to fit is seldom straight. En route, you'll probably experience different difficulties that test your purpose, flexibility, and responsibility. Understanding how to really explore these impediments is significant for supported progress and long haul achievement. This piece of the book is committed to recognizing normal difficulties in a change excursion and offering procedures to conquer them, beginning with perhaps of the most putting experience down: hitting a level.

Chapter 10: Dealing with Plateaus

Levels are a typical, though baffling, part of any weight reduction venture. They happen when progress, whether in weight reduction, strength gains, or wellness levels, appears to slow down in spite of keeping up with your eating routine and exercise routine. This section gives bits of knowledge into why levels occur and significant procedures to get through them, reigniting your advancement.

Figuring out Levels:

•Why Levels Happen: Investigating the physiological and metabolic variations that happen in light of weight reduction and expanded wellness, prompting levels. Understanding that levels are an indication of your body's productivity and variation.

•Perceiving a Genuine Level: Separating between a genuine level and ordinary variances in weight and wellness progress. Rules for recognizing when you've hit a level.

Systems for Conquering Levels:

•Reevaluating Your Propensities: Investigating your eating regimen and work-out daily practice to recognize likely regions for change. The significance of following admission and action levels precisely.

•Changing Your Caloric Admission: Tips for recalibrating your calorie needs founded on your ongoing weight and action level, as your energy prerequisites decline as you shed pounds.

•Fluctuating Your Work-out Everyday practice: The advantages of changing your gym routine to challenge your body in new ways, including adjusting force, span, and sort of activity.

•Expanding Bulk: How building muscle can assist with getting through weight reduction levels by expanding your basal metabolic rate, with systems for integrating strength preparing into your everyday practice.

Mental Parts of Levels:

•Overseeing Dissatisfaction and Remaining Propelled: Survival techniques for managing the profound effect of a level. Keeping sight of the headway made and keeping up with inspiration.

•Setting New, Non-Weight-Related Objectives: Zeroing in on execution, wellness, or wellbeing objectives that aren't attached to the scale to keep up with inspiration and pride.

When to Look for Proficient Assistance:

•Talking with a Nutritionist or Fitness coach: Conditions under which proficient exhortation can help recognize and defeat hindrances in your eating routine or exercise plan.

•Clinical Assessment: Taking into account a clinical assessment to preclude fundamental issues that could add to a level, like hormonal lopsided characteristics or metabolic circumstances.

Goals:

Toward the finish of this section, you'll comprehend that levels are a typical and regular piece of the change cycle. All the more critically, you'll be outfitted with various procedures to conquer them, guaranteeing proceeded with progress towards your fat-to-fit venture.

Focus point:

Levels are not an indication of disappointment but rather an encouragement to reevaluate and recalibrate your methodology. With the right changes and attitude, you can get through levels, find out about your body, and forge ahead with your way to enduring wellness and wellbeing.

Chapter 11: Managing Relapses

In the excursion from fat to fit, backslides — times when old propensities reemerge, prompting a brief inversion underway — are normal. Understanding how to deal with these minutes actually is urgent for long haul achievement and versatility. This section tends to why backslides occur and gives techniques to exploring them, guaranteeing they become opportunities for growth instead of hindrances.

Grasping Backslides:

•Why Backslides Happen: Investigating the mental and situational triggers that can prompt backslides, like pressure, personal disturbances, or critical life altering events. Perceiving that backslides are essential for the human experience and not characteristic of disappointment.

•Distinguishing Your Triggers: Methods for perceiving individual triggers and cautioning signs that a backslide might be inevitable, empowering preplanned activity.

Methodologies for Overseeing Backslides:

•Quick Reaction: How to successfully answer in the prompt consequence of a backslide, including tolerating what occurred, staying away from responsibility and self-fault, and pulling together on your objectives.

•Appraisal and Picking up: Assessing the conditions that prompted the backslide, what might have been done another way, and how to reinforce your system pushing ahead.

•Refocusing: Reasonable strides for continuing your solid propensities, whether it includes getting back to your work-out daily practice, committing once again to your nourishment plan, or both.

Building Strength:

•Reinforcing Resolution and Discipline: Methods for improving your discretion and discipline, like setting more modest, steady objectives and commending victories en route.

•Creating Survival methods: Laying out sound ways of dealing with hardship or stress for managing pressure and feelings, diminishing the probability of future backslides.

Keeping up with Long haul Achievement:

•Adaptable Mentality: Developing an outlook that embraces adaptability and versatility, considering changes in your arrangement on a case by case basis without review them as disappointments.

•Emotionally supportive network Use: Utilizing your emotionally supportive network during and after a backslide for consolation, responsibility, and guidance.

•Constant Objective Reconsideration: The significance of intermittently reevaluating your objectives to guarantee they stay reasonable and spurring.

Targets:

Toward the finish of this section, you'll perceive backslides as a component of the learning and development process. Furnished with techniques for overseeing them, you can limit their effect and arise more grounded, more proficient, and more dedicated to your excursion.

Focus point:

Backslides are not the finish of your change process yet a vital piece of the cycle. By grasping your triggers, answering helpfully, and involving each insight as an amazing chance to learn, you can construct flexibility and keep advancing toward your definitive objective of enduring wellness and wellbeing.

Chapter 12: The Role of Mindfulness and Stress Management

As we explore the intricacies of changing from fat to fit, the significance of mental and profound prosperity couldn't possibly be more significant. Stress and an absence of care can wreck your wellness objectives as well as effect your general wellbeing. This part digs into the job of care and successful pressure the board procedures, offering apparatuses to improve your change process both genuinely and intellectually.

Grasping the Effect of Pressure:

•Stress and Weight The executives: How persistent pressure can prompt weight gain through hormonal uneven characters (like expanded cortisol levels), profound eating, and disturbed rest designs.

•Stress and Exercise Execution: The impact of weight on inspiration, energy levels, and recuperation, featuring the significance of overseeing pressure for ideal activity execution.

Presenting Care:

•The Nuts and bolts of Care: An outline of care as the act of being completely present and participated in the occasion, mindful of your viewpoints and sentiments without interruption or judgment.

•Care for Wellbeing and Wellness: Investigating how care can work on dietary decisions, upgrade practice execution, and backing generally speaking prosperity by decreasing pressure, expanding center, and advancing a positive relationship with your body.

Care Practices:

•Careful Eating: Strategies for applying care to eating, empowering a better relationship with food, better processing, and more prominent fulfillment with dinners.

•Care Contemplation: Basic reflection practices to lessen pressure, work on close to home guideline, and improve mindfulness, including directed contemplations, breathing activities, and body filters.

•Integrating Care into Exercise: Methodologies for being more careful during active work to work on the nature of activity, increment satisfaction, and forestall injury.

Stress The board Procedures:

•Distinguishing Stressors: Apparatuses for perceiving and tending to the wellsprings of stress in your life, whether they're connected with work, connections, or individual assumptions.

•Successful Survival methods: A scope of procedures for overseeing pressure, from actual work and unwinding strategies to social help and time usage abilities.

•Making a Pressure Versatile Way of life: Ways to fabricate a way of life that innately decreases pressure, including laying out a daily practice, focusing on rest, and putting forth sensible objectives.

The Significance of Taking care of oneself:

•Taking care of oneself for Supportability: The job of taking care of oneself in keeping up with mental and actual wellbeing, forestalling burnout, and guaranteeing the manageability of your change endeavors.

•Taking care of oneself Practices: Ideas for taking care of oneself exercises that help pressure the board and care, like investing energy in nature, participating in leisure activities, and rehearsing appreciation.

Goals:

Toward the finish of this section, you'll comprehend the basic job that care and stress the board play in your change process. Furnished with useful devices and procedures, you can improve your psychological and profound prosperity, supporting your actual objectives.

Focal point:

Care and compelling pressure the board are not only valuable to your wellness process; they are basic components that help each part of your change. By incorporating these practices into your day to day routine, you can explore the difficulties of progress no sweat, strength, and achievement, guaranteeing an all encompassing way to deal with wellbeing and wellness.

5

Beyond Physical Transformation

As you approach the climax of your excursion from fat to fit, it's fundamental to perceive that genuine change rises above actual changes. Part V of this book centers around the significant effect of your excursion on close to home prosperity, self-improvement, and life viewpoint. Starting with close to home prosperity, this part investigates how accomplishing wellness objectives impacts and is affected by your profound wellbeing, giving procedures to supporting mental and profound equilibrium.

Chapter 13: Emotional Well-being

The association between actual wellness and close to home prosperity is certain. As you've attempted to change your body, you've probably experienced shifts in your close to home state, confidence, and generally life fulfillment. This section digs into the significance of profound prosperity in supporting your change and improving your personal satisfaction.

Grasping Profound Prosperity:

•The Connection Among Physical and Profound Wellbeing: Investigating how upgrades in actual wellbeing add to close to home soundness, stress decrease, and a positive mental self portrait.

•Perceiving Profound Changes: Recognizing normal close to home reactions to actual change, including expanded certainty, bliss in accomplishments, and now and then startling difficulties, for example, self-perception concerns.

Sustaining Profound Wellbeing:

•Self-Acknowledgment and Self esteem: Procedures for encouraging a solid relationship with yourself, recognizing your value past actual appearance, and commending your body for its capacities instead of simply its looks.

•Managing Profound Vacillations: Instruments for dealing with the close to home ups and downs that can go with huge way of life changes, including procedures for tending to negative self-talk and improving self-sympathy.

Upgrading Close to home Flexibility:

•Building Versatility: Methods for creating close to home strength, empowering you to confront future difficulties with strength and elegance, including the significance of adaptability, hopefulness, and the capacity to look for and acknowledge support.

•Survival techniques: Successful ways of dealing with stress for managing pressure, mishaps, and pessimistic feelings, zeroing in on solid outlets like imaginative articulation, social associations, and active work.

Supporting Close to home Prosperity:

•Care and Close to home Guideline: The job of care in keeping up with profound equilibrium, including rehearses that assist with remaining present and grounded.

•Nonstop Close to home Development: Empowering continuous self-improvement and profound development through self-reflection, acquiring new abilities, and taking part in exercises that give pleasure and satisfaction.

The More extensive Effect of Close to home Prosperity:

•Connections and Public activity: How further developed profound prosperity upgrades connections, correspondence, and social cooperations, adding to a more extravagant, more associated life.

•Life Fulfillment and Reason: The impact of close to home wellbeing on generally speaking life fulfillment, reason, and the quest for objectives past actual wellness.

Goals:

Toward the finish of this section, you will see the value in the basic job of close to home prosperity in your change process. Outfitted with methodologies to sustain your close to home wellbeing, you can keep up with the equilibrium important to partake in the full advantages of your actual accomplishments.

Action item:

Your excursion from fat to fit is as much about profound change for what it's worth about actual change. By focusing on profound prosperity, you improve not just your capacity to support your wellness accomplishments yet in addition your ability for bliss, versatility, and a profoundly fulfilling life.

Chapter 14: A New Perspective on Life

The excursion from fat to fit frequently prompts significant movements in your actual appearance, yet in your point of view, values, and needs. As you reshape your body, you likewise start to reshape your life, finding new interests, embracing difficulties, and survey the world from a perspective of probability and strengthening. This part investigates the extraordinary effect on your point of view of life, offering experiences into how to saddle these progressions for proceeded with development and satisfaction.

Finding Another Self-Personality:

•Past Actual Changes: Considering how the change venture reshapes your self-personality, moving from self inflicted constraints to an outlook of development and self-viability.

•Embracing Your Advanced Character: Procedures for incorporating your new mental self portrait into your feeling of personality, recognizing the strength, discipline, and versatility you've created.

Extended Skylines and New Interests:

•Investigating New Interests: Empowering the investigation of interests and exercises that your past way of life might have blocked, from outside undertakings to serious games, and how these can additionally advance your life.

•Deep rooted Learning: The significance of staying open to realizing, whether it's connected with wellness, sustenance, or altogether new fields. Embracing a mentality of interest and nonstop improvement.

Changes in Connections and Social Elements:

•Exploring Movements in Connections: Understanding what your change could mean for associations with companions, family, and partners. Systems for encouraging steady, positive associations and managing likely difficulties.

•Fabricating New People group: The job of new interests and way of life changes in driving you to new networks and groups of friends that share your qualities and objectives.

A More profound Appreciation for Wellbeing and Prosperity:

•Esteeming Wellbeing Past Style: Moving concentration from simply stylish objectives to a more profound appreciation for wellbeing, prosperity, and practical wellness, perceiving the more extensive advantages of your way of life changes.

•Advancing a Culture of Wellbeing: How your process can move and impact others around you to focus on their wellbeing, going about as a good example and supporter for a solid, dynamic way of life.

Living Deliberately:

•Settling on Cognizant Decisions: The change venture as an illustration in pursuing purposeful decisions about how you live, from everyday propensities to life objectives, adjusting your activities to your qualities and yearnings.

•The Force of Objectives: Proceeding to put forth and seek after objectives, both inside and past the domain of wellness, as a method for driving self-awareness and satisfaction.

Confronting the Future with Certainty:

•Embracing Vulnerability: Building the certainty to confront life's vulnerabilities and difficulties, outfitted with the information that you have the strength and versatility to defeat obstructions.

•A Forward-Looking Outlook: Developing a hopeful, forward-looking mentality that spotlights on potential and conceivable outcomes, instead of limits.

Targets:

Toward the finish of this part, you'll perceive the way your change process has gifted you with another point of view on life. This freshly discovered standpoint enables you to seek after an existence of direction, energy, and constant development.

Important point:

The excursion from fat to fit is extraordinary in manners that reach out a long ways past the physical. An odyssey difficulties and changes you, offering another point of view on life that values development, wellbeing, and satisfaction. As you push ahead, outfitted with this new viewpoint, you are more ready to make every moment count, embracing each a valuable open door for satisfaction and achievement.

Chapter 15: Maintaining Your Transformation

The last part of your excursion from fat to fit isn't an end, yet entirely a fresh start. Keeping up with your change is tied in with coordinating the examples learned, propensities shaped, and qualities acquired into a feasible way of life that keeps on supporting your wellbeing and bliss. This section centers around systems for supporting your physical, mental, and close to home accomplishments, guaranteeing that the progressions you've made turned into a long-lasting piece of your life.

Way of life Mix:

•Maintainable Propensities: Underlining the significance of consistency in nourishment, exercise, and stress the executives rehearses. Ways to make solid propensities an easy aspect of your everyday daily practice.

•Versatility: How to stay adaptable and adjust your propensities as your life altering events, guaranteeing that your way of life keeps on supporting your wellbeing objectives.

Consistent Objective Setting:

•Putting forth New Objectives: The job of setting new, testing, however reachable objectives to keep yourself roused and participated in your wellbeing process.

•Expanding Your Perspectives: Empowering objectives past actual wellness, for example, self-awareness, vocation aspirations, or mastering new abilities, to advance by and large life fulfillment and satisfaction.

Outlook for Long haul Achievement:

•Development Mentality: Developing an outlook that embraces difficulties, gains from misfortunes, and perspectives exertion as a way to dominance.

•Self-Sympathy and Absolution: Perceiving the significance of self-empathy notwithstanding mishaps. Understanding that mistakes are essential for the excursion and not characteristic of disappointment.

Local area and Backing:

•Utilizing Encouraging groups of people: The significance of keeping up with and growing your encouraging group of people, including family, companions, and networks that share your qualities and objectives.

•Turning into a Good example: How your process can move others. The advantages of sharing your story and encounters to inspire and uphold everyone around you.

Wellbeing as a Long lasting Excursion:

•Past the Physical: Recognizing that genuine wellbeing envelops physical, mental, and profound prosperity, and focusing on sustaining all parts of your wellbeing.

•Deep rooted Learning and Investigation: Remaining inquisitive and open to new encounters, whether connected with wellbeing and wellness or different areas of individual premium.

Confronting Future Difficulties:

•Expecting and Conquering Obstructions: Systems for expecting future difficulties and arranging how to explore them, building up the strength you've constructed.

•Observing Your Excursion: Consistently considering and praising the headway you've made, recognizing the work and commitment it took to change your life.

Targets:

Toward the finish of this section, you will have a diagram for keeping up with your change and proceeding to develop and flourish. You'll comprehend that supporting your new way of life is a unique cycle that requires continuous responsibility, versatility, and self-reflection.

Focal point:

Keeping up with your change is about more than saving the actual changes you've accomplished; it's tied in with living in arrangement with your freshly discovered values, consistently putting forth and chasing after objectives, and contributing decidedly to your local area. Your excursion from fat to fit has furnished you with the devices, information, and strength expected to explore the way forward, guaranteeing that your best self is consistently reachable.

Conclusion

As we arrive at the finish of "Fat to Fit: Change Your Body, Change Your Life," it's critical to stop and ponder the excursion we've embraced together. From the underlying strides of understanding your body and the study of weight gain, through laying out reasonable objectives and planning intellectually for change, to embracing the change venture and defeating difficulties, every section has been a stage toward a significant individual change — genuinely, yet intellectually and sincerely too.

Summing up Key Important points:

•The All encompassing Way to deal with Change: Genuine change includes a complete methodology that incorporates physical, mental, and close to home wellbeing. It's about something other than shedding pounds or getting fit; it's tied in with upgrading your general personal satisfaction.

•Maintainable Change Comes from The inside: Enduring change is established in a profound comprehension of oneself, a guarantee to supportable propensities, and an outlook designed for development and strength.

•The Force of Local area and Backing: No excursion ought to be attempted alone. The help of companions, family, and similar people is significant in keeping up with inspiration and defeating difficulties.

•Deep rooted Excursion: Change isn't an objective yet a persistent excursion of development and self-disclosure. It requires continuous responsibility, flexibility, and a readiness to confront new difficulties with boldness and positive thinking.

Empowering Long lasting Wellbeing and Health:

Your process doesn't end here. The practices, bits of knowledge, and propensities you've created are the establishment for a long period of wellbeing and health. Ceaselessly laying out new objectives, investigating new interests, and developing a steady local area are fundamental systems for supporting your change.

Keep in mind, wellbeing and health are not static; they adjust as you travel through various phases of life. Embracing this development with an open heart and an inquisitive brain will guarantee that your process isn't recently supported yet improved.

Last Encouraging statements:

As you push ahead, equipped with the information, encounters, and methodologies you've acquired, realize that you have the ability to significantly impact your life as per your most profound qualities and most elevated goals. Your change process is a demonstration of your solidarity, strength, and limit with respect to change.

Let your excursion from fat to fit be a signal for other people who try to leave on their own ways of change. Share your story, loan your help, and keep on rousing.

Most importantly, appreciate the excursion. Every day offers another amazing chance to develop, to challenge yourself, and to completely live. Embrace these open doors with energy and appreciation, realizing that your best self is certainly not a decent ideal however a skyline that grows as you approach it.

Congrats on all you have accomplished and all that is on the way. Here's to your wellbeing, your joy, and your proceeded with change.